Why We Eat Protein

by Beth Bence Reinke, MS, RD

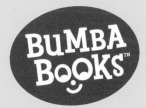

BUMBA BOOKS™

LERNER PUBLICATIONS ◆ MINNEAPOLIS

Note to Educators:

Throughout this book, you'll find critical thinking questions. These can be used to engage young readers in thinking critically about the topic and in using the text and photos to do so.

Lerner Publications Company
A division of Lerner Publishing Group, Inc.
241 First Avenue North
Minneapolis, MN 55401 USA

For reading levels and more information, look up this title at www.lernerbooks.com.

Library of Congress Cataloging-in-Publication Data

Names: Reinke, Beth Bence, author.
Title: Why we eat protein / Beth Bence Reinke, MS, RD.
Description: Minneapolis : Lerner Publications, [2018] | Series: Bumba books. Nutrition matters | Audience: Ages 4–7. | Audience: K to grade 3. | Includes bibliographical references and index.
Identifiers: LCCN 2017047423 (print) | LCCN 2017057715 (ebook) | ISBN 9781541507722 (eb pdf) | ISBN 9781541503397 (lb : alk. paper) | ISBN 9781541526853 (pb : alk. paper)
Subjects: LCSH: Proteins in human nutrition—Juvenile literature. | Proteins—Juvenile literature.
Classification: LCC TX553.P7 (ebook) | LCC TX553.P7 R45 2018 (print) | DDC 613.2/82—dc23

LC record available at https://lccn.loc.gov/2017047423

Manufactured in the United States of America
1 – CG – 7/15/18

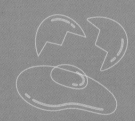

Table of Contents

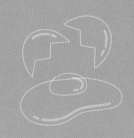

All about Protein

Eating protein helps you grow.

It helps make your body strong.

Did you eat protein today?

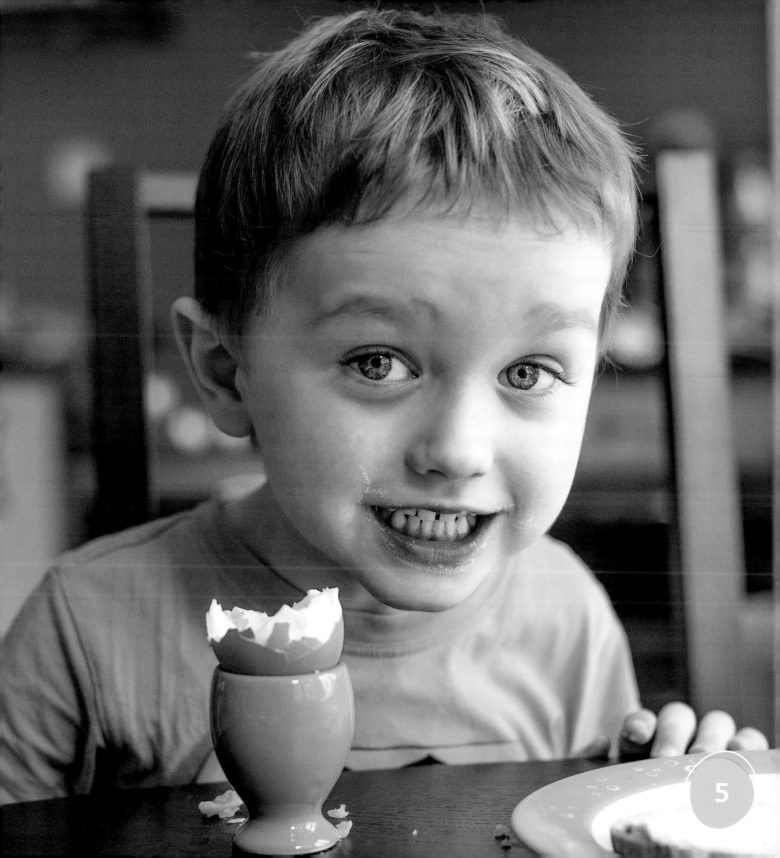

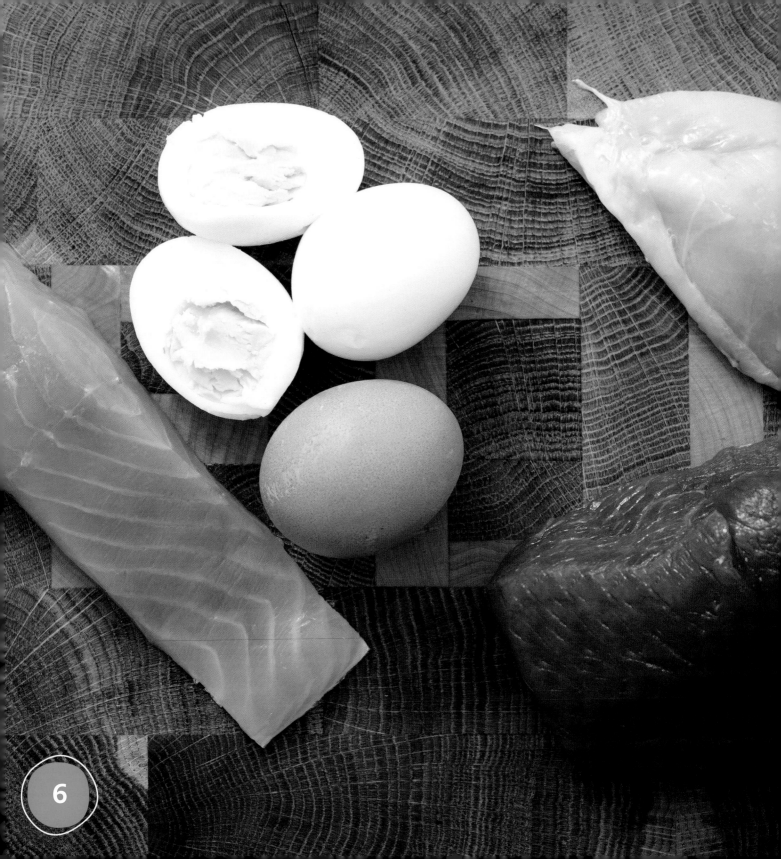

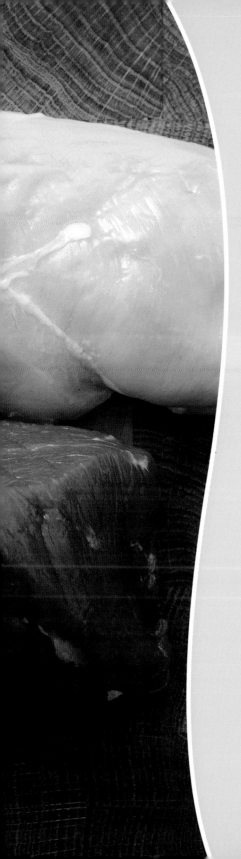

Animal foods are rich

in protein.

Meat and poultry

have protein.

So do fish and eggs.

Some plant foods have protein.

Beans are one of these.

Nuts and seeds have protein too.

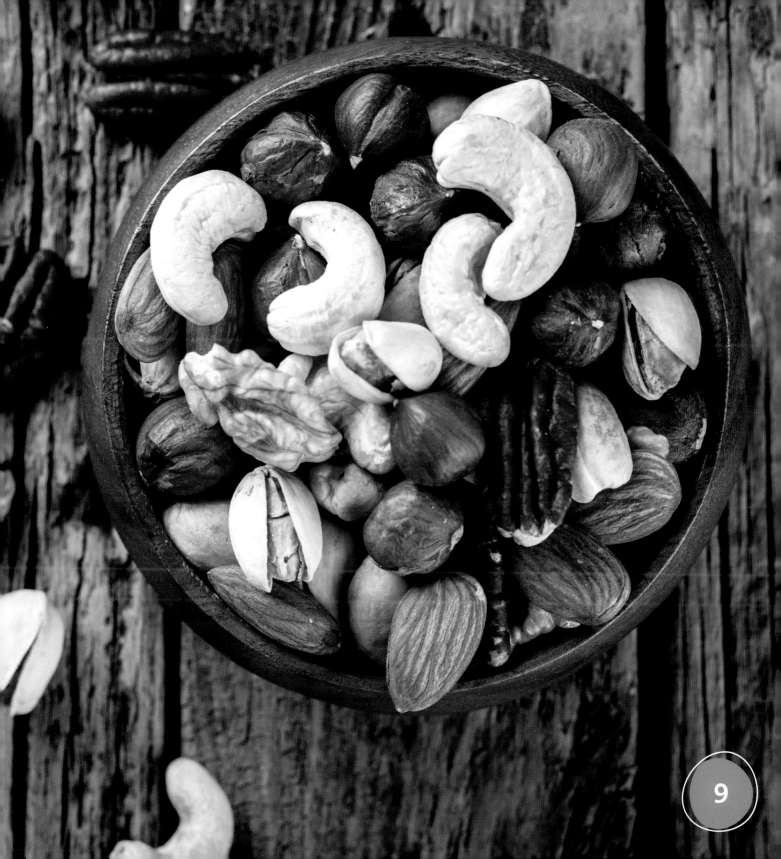

Protein keeps your bones healthy.

It helps you build strong muscles.

Why do you think you need healthy bones?

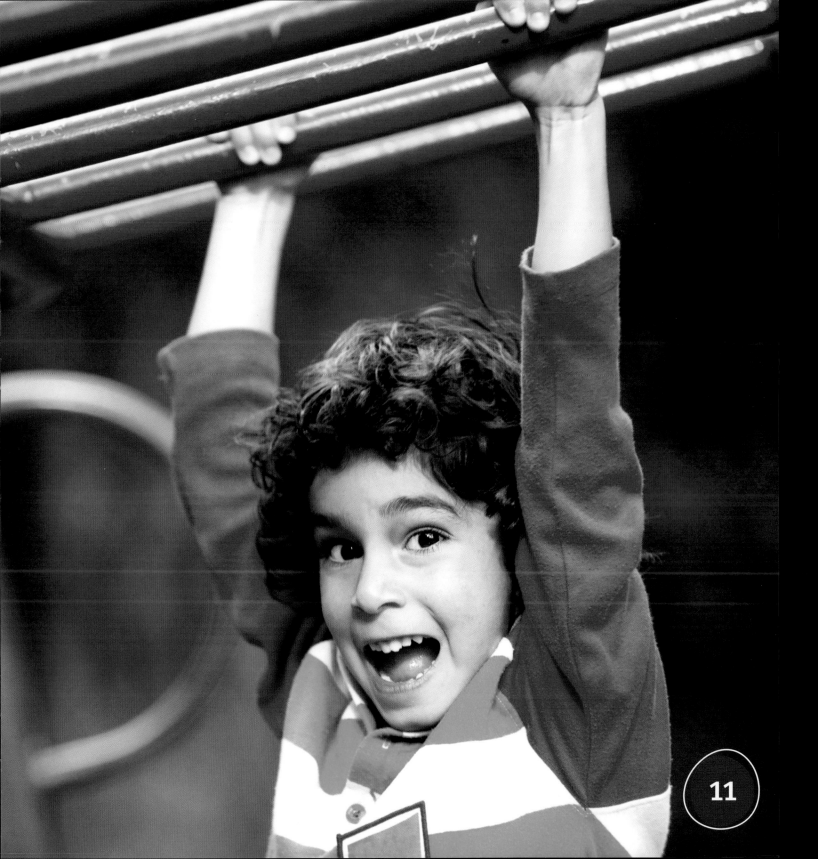

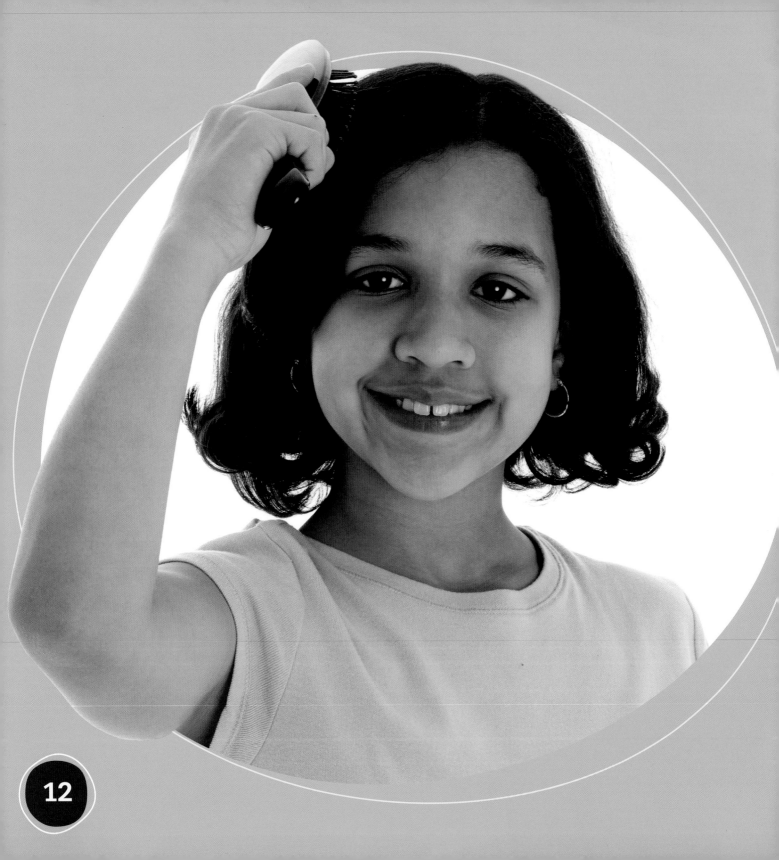

You need protein to grow hair
and make skin.

Eating protein helps your body
make blood.

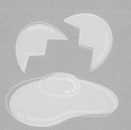

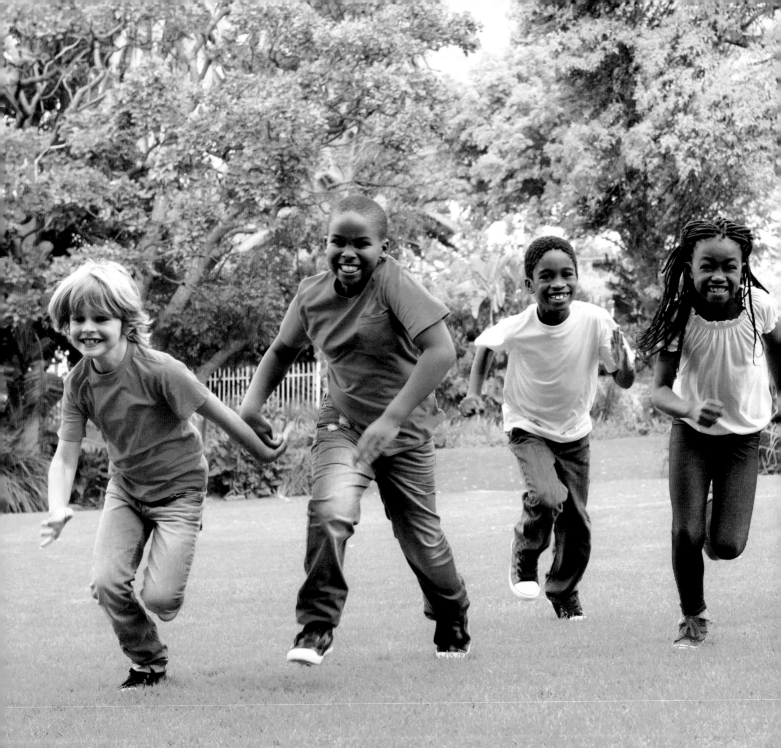

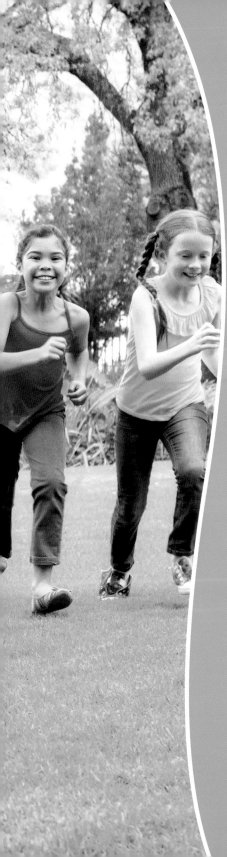

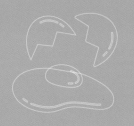

Iron is a mineral in protein foods.

Iron helps your body use oxygen.

How do you think your body uses oxygen?

15

B vitamins are in protein foods.

B vitamins give you energy to play and grow.

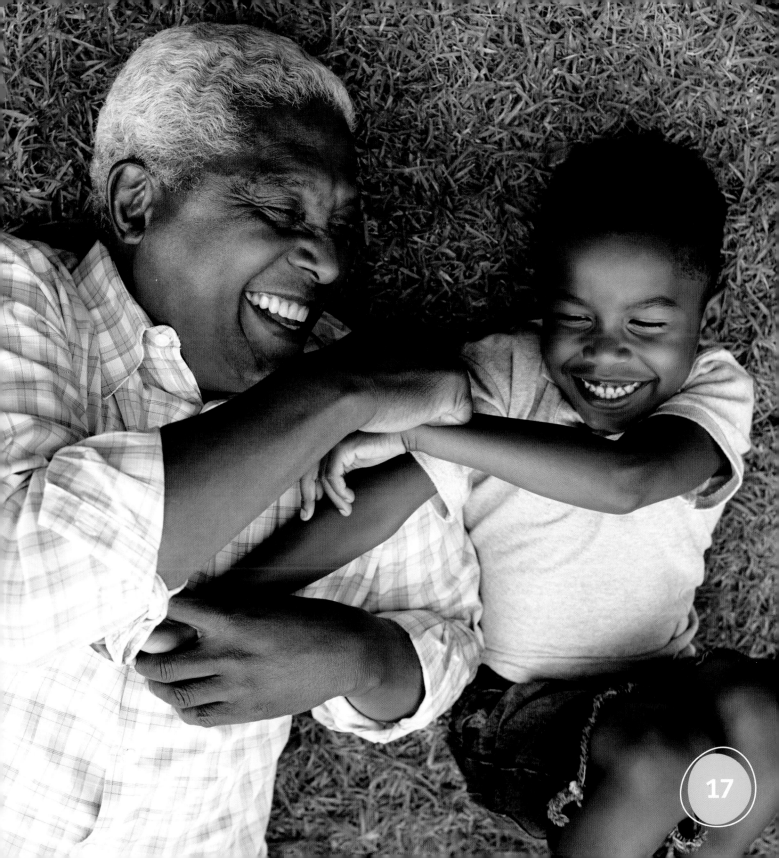

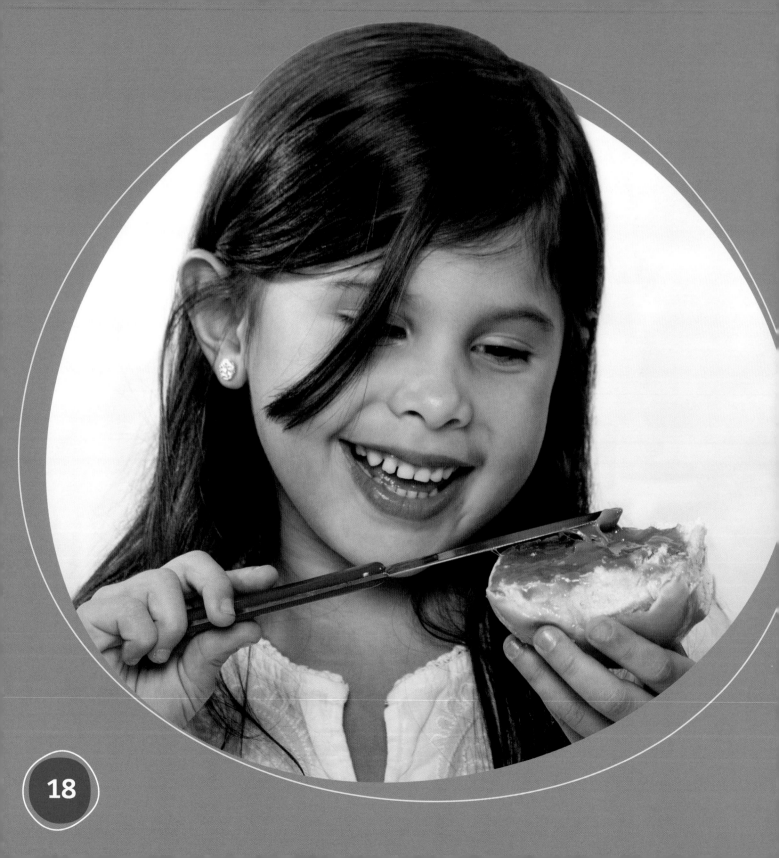

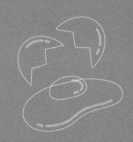

You need four servings of protein

each day.

One egg is a serving.

So is a spoonful of peanut butter.

What protein foods did you eat today?

Eating protein helps you stay healthy.

What are your favorite protein foods?

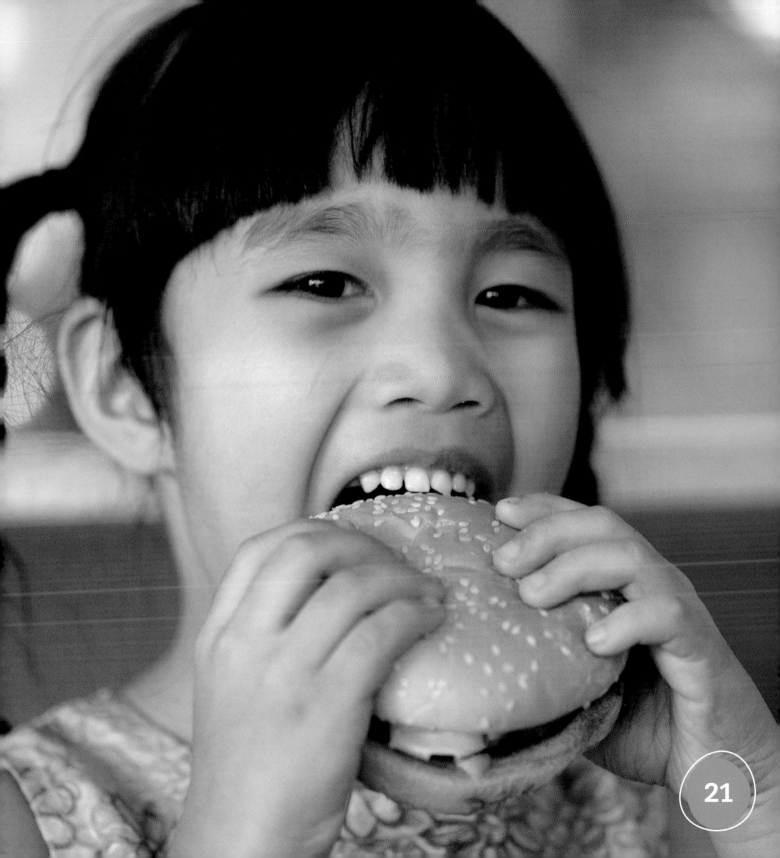

USDA MyPlate Diagram

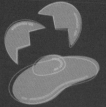

Fill this much of your plate with protein foods.

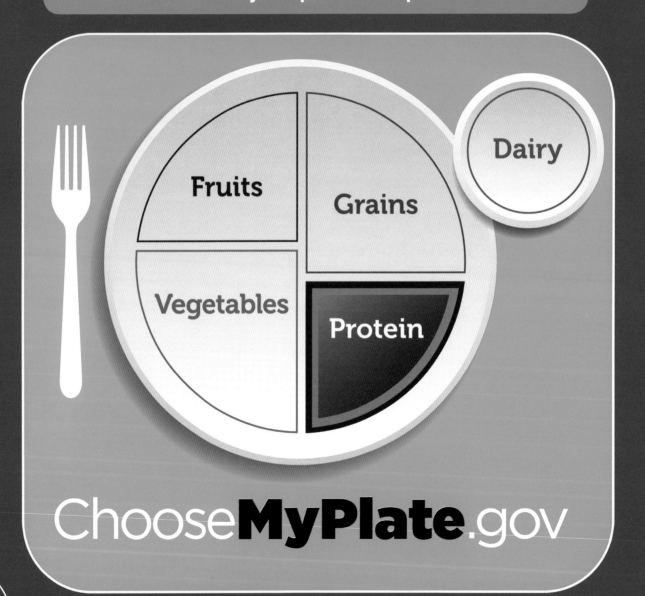

Picture Glossary

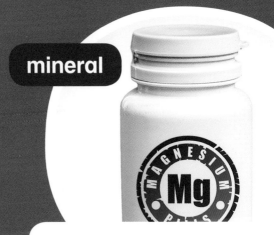

mineral

a nutrient such as iron, zinc, and others that your body needs for good health

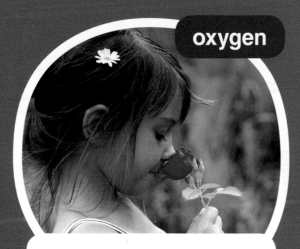

oxygen

a gas that we breathe in and that the body needs to live

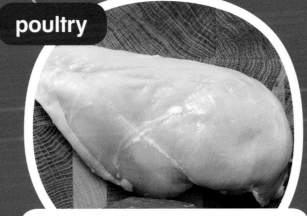

poultry

meat from birds such as chickens and turkeys

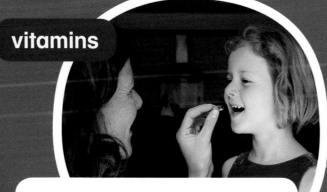

vitamins

nutrients such as vitamin A, vitamin C, and others that your body needs for good health

23

Read More

Black, Vanessa. *Protein Foods*. Minneapolis: Jump!, 2017.

Borgert-Spaniol, Megan. *Protein Foods Group*. Minneapolis: Bellwether Media, 2012.

Parker, Victoria. *All about Meat and Fish*. Irvine, CA: QEB, 2009.

Index

Photo Credits